SMOOTHIE RECIPES

Tastiest Smoothie Recipes (Green Smoothies, Smoothies for Weight Loss, Smoothie Cleanse, Detox Smoothies, Smoothie Diet, Energy Smoothies)

Introduction

If you are someone who's concerned about living a healthy lifestyle by ensuring that you get your daily dose of fruits and vegetables, then it will no longer come as a surprise if you have already heard about smoothies. These are healthy and delicious drinks that will let you include more fruits and vegetables into your diet. You can get more than half of your daily nutrition needs in just a glass. You can also gain several health benefits such as better energy, healthier organs and weight loss.

Smoothies are easy to make. All you need is a blender and basic kitchen tools such as knife and cutting board. You don't have to be an expert in the kitchen to whip up delicious smoothie.

Read this book today and find out how to make delicious, healthy smoothies in just a few minutes.

Table of Contents

Chapter 1: Green Smoothies

Green smoothies are rich in fiber, minerals and vitamins. These drinks also allow you to add more vegetables in your daily diet. These smoothies use green vegetables as the main ingredients; hence, the color, but you can also add other colored fruits and vegetables such as pears, bananas, seeds, nuts, etc.

Macha Pear Green Smoothie

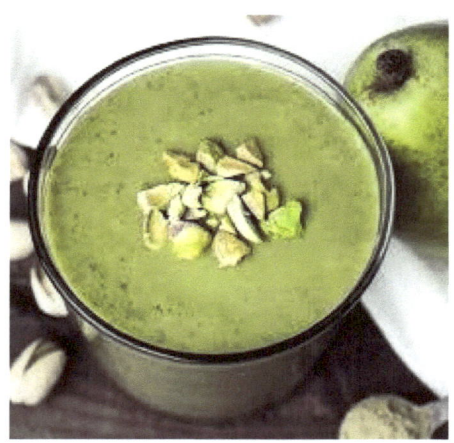

Macha is fast becoming a popular drink. It is chock-full of antioxidants that help in detoxifying the body, removing free radicals and protecting it against oxidative damage and a host of other health benefits.

In this recipe, macha supplies your body with caffeine, which boosts your energy and improves your focus. Spinach provides almost all of the important nutrients that your body needs. Pear is added to sweeten the smoothie. Not only that, pear also adds more fiber and Vitamin C to this powerful drink. When adding pear, keep the skin on. This is where you can find most of the important phytonutrients.

Ingredients

- 2 scoops protein powder, vanilla flavor
- 1/2 teaspoon of macha tea powder
- 1 cup unsweetened almond milk
- 1 pear, cored 1 cup spinach

To prepare:

It is easy to make this nutritious green smoothie. All you have to do is to prepare all the ingredients, put in a blender and pulse on medium speed. When the mixture becomes smooth and creamy, transfer it into your glass and enjoy.

Nutritional Facts

In a 16-ounce serving, you'll get:

- 299 calories
- 37 g carbohydrates
- 27 g sugar
- 6 g fat (2 g saturated)
- 9 g fiber
- 595 mg sodium
- 27 g protein

Orange Kale Green Smoothie

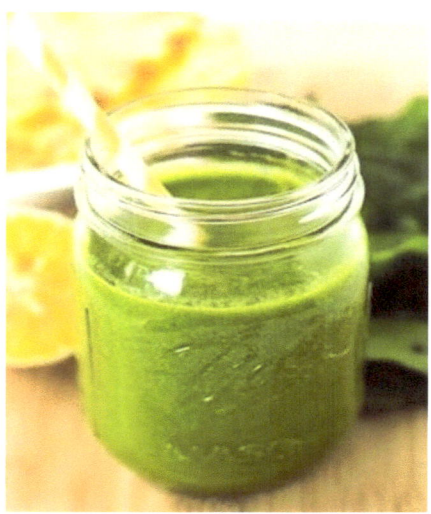

This green smoothie is a one-two punch drink. It energizes your body while detoxifying it. This recipe contains a lot of proteins and provides you with all the nutrients you need for an energy-filled day.

Fresh orange and spirulina, when combined, can produce a drink filled with fiber, Vitamin C, beta-carotene and iron. Protein is at 30 grams, all from plants. This will keep your muscles happy, especially if you drink this after an intense workout.

Ingredients:

- 2 scoops protein powder, vanilla flavor
- 1 orange, peel and seeds removed
- 1 cup chopped raw kale
- 1/2 teaspoon of spirulina powder
- 1 pinch of ginger powder
- 1 pinch of ground cinnamon
- 1 cup water

To prepare:

Measure the ingredients and place in a blender. Pulse until smooth.

Nutritional Facts:

Per 16-ounce serving:

- 300 calories
- 35 g carbohydrates
- 23 g sugar
- 7 g fiber
- 6 g fat (2 g saturated fats)
- 30 g protein
- 613 mg sodium

Peach Green Smoothie

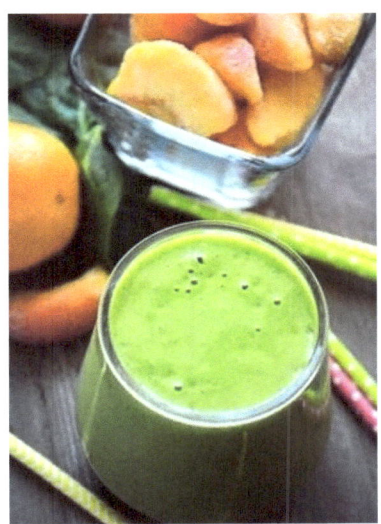

This is quick and easy to make. You can make this to power up your day. Keep a serving handy.

Peaches are full of antioxidants with a long list of benefits including its anti-cancer, anti-inflammatory and anti-aging effects. Banana is high in potassium, which helps your muscles function better. You also have pineapples with bromelain, which prevents inflammation and offers cardiovascular support.

Don't forget the benefits you'll get from flaxseeds, a rich source of healthy fats. Expect to feel full from just a glass of this healthy, delicious smoothie. The protein boost comes from the protein powder. The vanilla flavor helps in releasing the delicious flavors of the fruits.

Ingredients:

- 1 cup unsweetened almond milk
- 2 scoops vanilla protein powder
- 2 cups kale
- 1/2 cup frozen pineapple
- 1 cup frozen peaches
- 1/2 banana
- 1 tablespoon ground flaxseed

To prepare:

Place all the ingredients in a blender. Blend until smooth.

Nutritional Facts:

Per 20-ounce serving:

- 436 calories
- 62 g carbohydrates
- 33 g protein
- 9 g fat (2.5 g saturated)

- 629 mg sodium

Minty Cucumber and Apple Smoothie

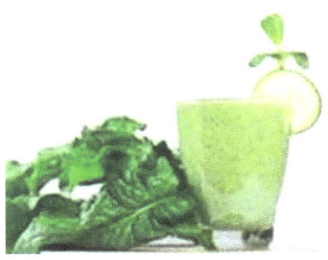

Not all green smoothies contain leafy greens. Some recipes actually use both fruits and vegetables as their main ingredients. Take a look at this recipe.

Cucumber makes this green smoothie rich in vitamins and minerals. It also gives its refreshing flavor. Mint also adds to the refreshing effect of this fruity green smoothie. It helps improve digestion and promote better metabolism. Apple gives the sweet fruity flavor. The juice concentrate is full of natural sugars, thereby ensuring that you won't deal with the negative effects of refined sugar. It is all-natural and good for your health.

Ingredients:

- 1/3 cup unsweetened 100% apple juice concentrate, undiluted
- 1 cup cucumber, peel and seeds removed then chopped
- 1/4 cup chopped fresh mint leaves
- 1/4 cup cold water
- 10 (about 4 ounces) ice cubes

Measure and place the ingredients in a blender. Blend until your desired smoothness is achieved. Transfer into your glass, so you can enjoy its refreshing fruity goodness.

Nutritional Facts:

- Calories 91
- Carbohydrate 21.6 g
- Fiber 1.4 g
- Fat 0.4 g
- Saturated fat 0.1 g
- Polyunsaturated fat 0.1 g
- Protein 1 g
- Iron 2 mg
- Calcium 41 mg
- Sodium 16 mg

Kiwi Green Apple Lime and Collard Green Smoothie

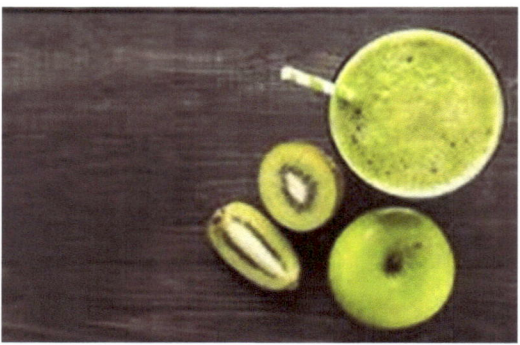

Everything is green in this fruit and vegetable combination. This smoothie improves your immune system and protects the body not just against infections, but from cancer-causing free radicals as well.

Kiwi, green apple and lime all give this recipe a refreshing taste, while collard gives it the goodness that only vegetables can bring. This is high in fiber, which promotes better digestive movement. Its high fiber content also ensures that toxins will be removed from your body. Vitamin C and other vitamins and minerals from the fruits and from collard promote better health.

Ingredients:

- 1 medium kiwi fruit, chopped
- ½ medium green apple, core removed and sliced
- ½ cup collard greens
- 2 tablespoon fresh lime juice
- water

To make:

Put all the sliced fruits and vegetable in a blender. Add lime juice. Pour enough water to cover everything. Puree until smooth. Pour in your glass and enjoy.

Nutritional Facts:

- 105 calories
- 26.6 g total carbohydrates
- 16.6 g sugars
- 5.3 g dietary fiber
- 0.7 g total fat
- 0 mg cholesterol
- 1.7 g protein
- 7 mg sodium

Guava and Kiwi with Coconut Smoothie

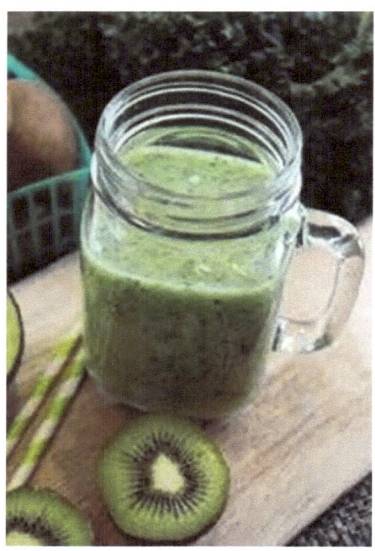

This simple green smoothie rich in nutrients that strengthen your immune system. It is rich in vitamins and minerals, as well as phytonutrients that can help fight cancer cells.

Guava contains Vitamin C, which strengthens your immunity and protects your body against free radicals. Kiwi is full of vitamins and minerals that help prevent cancer formation. Coconut gives this smoothie a creamy texture. It also provides a healthy dose of fats that help you feel full and satisfied with just a serving. Try this recipe today and experience its goodness.

Ingredients:

- 1 medium kiwi fruit, sliced
- 2/3 cup coconut water
- 1 medium guava, sliced

- ¼ cup crushed ice

To make:

Place all ingredients in a blender. Pulse until smooth and evenly blended. Pour in one glass, so you can start enjoying it.

Nutritional Facts:

- 138 calories
- 30 g total carbohydrates
- 19.0 g sugar
- 8.9 g dietary fiber
- 1.6 g total fat
- 0 mg cholesterol
- 4.3 g protein
- 172 mg sodium

Chapter 2: Detox Smoothies

Smoothies are perfect for quick and easy detox. These are easy to make, yet powerful since it works effectively in cleansing your system from within. Detoxing with smoothies is also a great way to remove harmful toxins from your body while also giving you a good supply of nutrients. Detoxifying your body shouldn't be a reason to deprive it with nutrients. You get optimum benefits from detox if you still make sure that your body is well-nourished during the process.

Super Kale Detox Green Smoothie

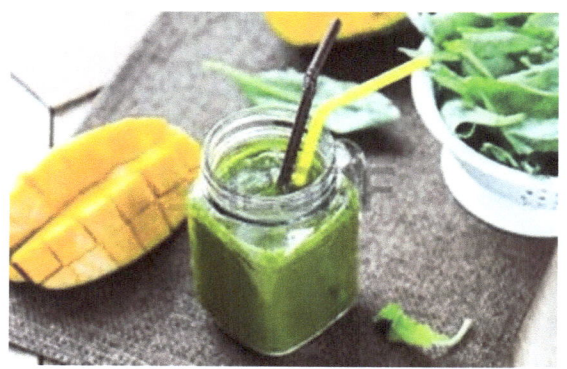

This is a powerful simple smoothie. The main ingredient, kale, is rich in nutrients such as magnesium, calcium, Vitamin C and large amounts of phytonutrients, to name a few.

Mango gives your smoothie a natural sweetness, which improves its taste. It is also full of fiber, minerals and vitamins that support better health. Parsley and celery add to the bright green color of the smoothie. These ingredients act as diuretics, promoting urination to excrete toxin from your body.

Ingredients (makes 2 servings):

- 1¼ cups chopped kale leaves (stems and tough rib removed)
- 2 medium ribs celery, chopped
- ¼ cup chopped flat-leaf parsley
- 1¼ cups frozen cubed mango
- 1 cup chilled fresh tangerine or orange juice
- ¼ cup chopped fresh mint

Mix all the ingredients in a blender and pulse on high speed until smooth and creamy.

Nutritional Facts:

Per serving:

- 160 calories
- 39 g carbohydrates
- 5 g fiber
- 3 g protein
- 0.5 g fat (0 g saturated fats)
- 56 mg sodium

Berry Detox Smoothie

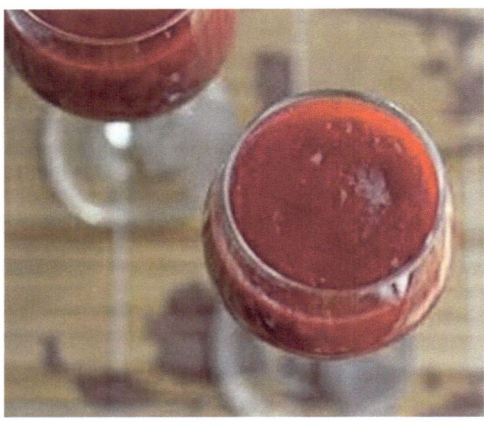

This smoothie has a beautiful pink shade, which is sure to entice you to drink more. More than its appetizing color, this smoothie is full of detoxifying enzymes that remove toxins from your body. The nutrients are also helpful in promoting better digestion, which further cleanses your body from within.

Berries are rich in phytonutrients that stimulate the detoxification process to start. These remove free radicals from the tissues and bring them out for excretion. Ginger gives the smoothie a little kick to offset the sweetness of the berries. It is also a great addition to the drink because it further improves the function of your digestive tract.

Ingredients (makes 2 servings):

- 1 cup frozen raspberries, unsweetened
- ¼ cup frozen unsweetened cherries (pitted) or raspberries
- ¾ cup chilled rice or almond milk, unsweetened
- 1 ½ tablespoon of honey
- 1 teaspoon of ground flaxseed

- 2 teaspoon of fresh ginger, finely grated
- 1-2 teaspoon of freshly squeezed lemon juice

Mix all of the ingredients in a blender. Adjust the amount of lemon juice based on the level of tartness that you want your smoothie to have. Blend until smooth and mixed well. Pour in your glass, then drink for better health.

Nutritional Facts (per serving):

- 112 calories
- 26 g carbohydrates
- 3 g fiber
- 1 g protein
- 1.5 g fat (0 g saturated fats)
- 56 mg sodium

5-Ingredient Detox Smoothie

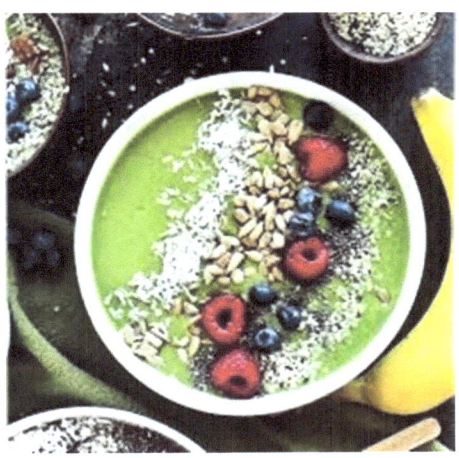

This simple smoothie is full of antioxidants and fiber. It is also rich in nutrients that boost your body's immune function. This will greatly help you in getting rid of the toxins that cause damage to your cells. Drink this for breakfast, so you can start the detoxification process early in the day. You can also take it for snacks to get toxins out of your system for the entire day.

You can choose a 5th ingredient (fruit juice) to make your own version of this smoothie. You can put freshly squeezed lime, lemon or orange juice. You may also put juice concentrates that you love, or you can mix juices and add them here as the 5th ingredient.

Ingredients (makes 2 servings):

- 1 cup organic spinach or kale
- 1 cup frozen berries
- 1 tablespoon flax seed meal
- 1/2 cup bananas, peeled, sliced & frozen
- 1 cup fruit juice of your choice

To make:

Put everything in a blender and blend using medium to high speed, until your preferred smoothness is reached. You may add more juice if you want a thinner consistency.

Nutritional Facts (per serving):

- 181 calories
- 41 g carbohydrates
- 4.7 g fiber
- 29 g sugar
- 1.6 g fat (0 g saturated fat)
- 2.5 g protein
- 19 mg sodium

Strawberry Kiwi Banana Smoothie

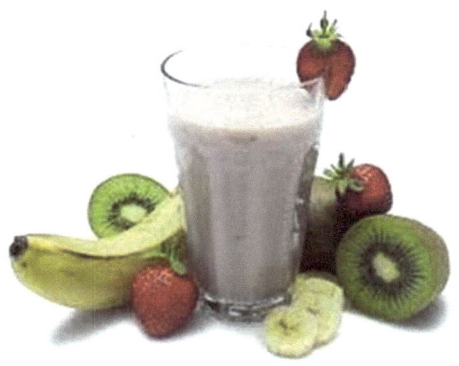

This is a refreshing smoothie, which also detoxifies your body. Kiwi, banana and strawberry supply your body with nutrients that help get rid of toxins while strengthening your tissues.

Kiwi and strawberry are abundant in Vitamin C, potassium and dietary fiber. Both these ingredients can also supply your body with iodine, Vitamin K, manganese, magnesium and folate. These minerals and vitamins promote good eye health and stronger bones. These also minimize inflammation in the body, have anti-cancer effects and protect the cardiovascular system.

Of course, there is banana with its excellent amount of potassium. Banana promotes better digestive function, regular waste elimination, improved bone health and better eye health. It also helps in preventing the development of cancer.

Ingredients:

- 1 cup water
- 1 kiwi, peeled and halved
- 1 cup fresh or frozen strawberries
- 1 fresh or frozen medium banana

- 1 teaspoon coconut oil
- 4-6 ice cubes

To make:

Simply put all the ingredients in a blender. Blend using medium speed until the mixture reaches your preferred smoothness. Pour in your glass and enjoy the health benefits all day long.

Nutritional Facts:

- Calories: 233
- Carbohydrates: 48g
- Sugar: 28g
- Fiber: 8g
- Fat: 6g
- Protein: 3g
- Vitamin C: 265% RDA
- Calcium: 6% RDA
- Vitamin K: 40% RDA
- Iron: 6% RDA

Green Tea with Spinach Lime and Apple Smoothie

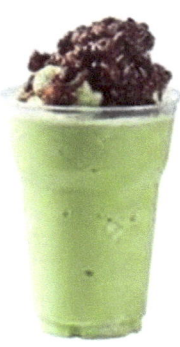

Green tea is an excellent ingredient, which you can add to make a powerful detox smoothie. It has an excellent amount of antioxidants that get rid of toxins and free radicals while protecting the cells from damage.

Spinach is rich in phytonutrients, minerals, fibers and vitamins that support detoxification. Lime gives this mix tartness, thereby enhancing its flavor. It is also a good source of Vitamin C, which acts as an antioxidant. Apple rounds up the flavor with its natural sweetness. Keep the peel on for more fiber and phytonutrients. All these ingredients will help you have regular bowel movements, which is necessary to remove wastes and toxins.

Ingredients:

- ¾ cup green tea
- 1 medium apple, sliced
- ½ cup shredded baby spinach
- 1 tablespoon lime juice

To make:

Place everything in a blender and pulse until smooth. Pour in a serving glass. You can garnish with an apple or lime wedge if you want.

Nutritional Facts:

- 102 calories
- 26.9 g carbohydrates
- 4.8 g dietary fiber
- 19.2 g sugar
- 0.4 g total fat
- O mg cholesterol

- 1.0 g protein
- 14 mg sodium

Cucumber Dill with Carrot and Orange Smoothie

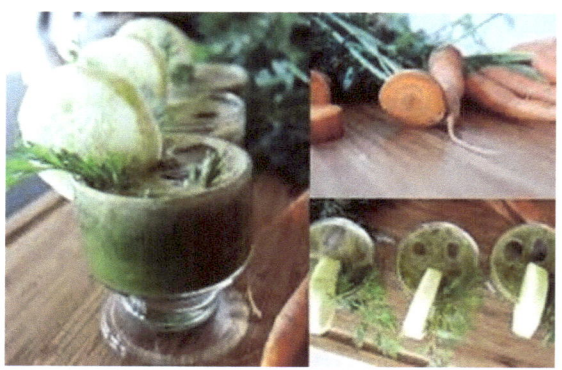

This is a refreshing way to detox your body. All the ingredients work together to promote the removal of toxins from the body regularly. Carrot is rich in beta-carotene, which is a potent group of natural plant chemicals with antioxidant actions. Dill is an excellent herb, which promotes better bowel movement necessary for toxin elimination. Orange and cucumber are rich in vitamins and minerals that further promote detoxification. All these combine to create a powerful and delicious way to detoxify.

Ingredients:

- ½ cup freshly squeezed orange juice
- ½ medium carrot, sliced
- 1 teaspoon dill weed

- ¼ medium cucumber, sliced
- water

To make:

Place the ingredients in a blender and puree until smooth. Add water to adjust the consistency to your liking. Pour in a glass and garnish with a cucumber slice or orange wedge.

Nutritional facts:

- 82 calories
- 19.2 g total carbohydrates
- 13.2 g sugars
- 1.5 g dietary fiber
- 0.4 g total fat
- 1.8 g protein
- 26 mg sodium

Cucumber Pistachio with Celery and Honey Smoothie

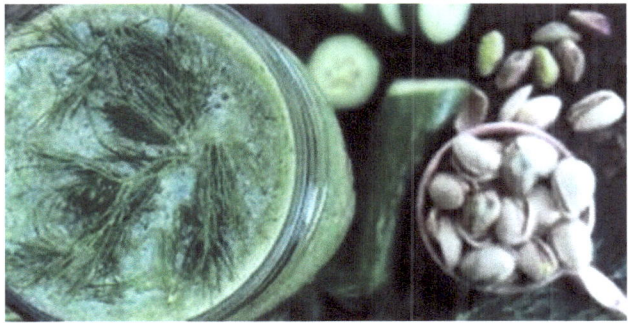

All the ingredients combine to form a smoothie, which promotes waste and toxin eradication. These contain nutrients that reduce inflammation, promote healing and help with tissue repair. The phytonutrients from these ingredients have potent antioxidant power, which effectively detoxifies the body.

Ingredients:

- 1 medium celery stalk, diced
- ½ medium cucumber, sliced
- 1 teaspoon honey
- 10 grams or a handful of pistachio nuts
- water to max line

To make:

Place the sliced fruits and vegetable in a blender. Pour enough water to cover all the ingredients. Blend until smooth. Pour in a tall glass and serve with crushed pistachios and a celery stalk. You can drizzle more honey if you want.

Nutritional Facts:

- 106 calories
- 15.2 g carbohydrates
- 9.6 g sugar
- 2.4 g dietary fiber
- 4.7 g total fat
- 3.3 g protein
- 35 mg sodium

Chapter 3: Protein Smoothies

Banana and Oats Protein Smoothie

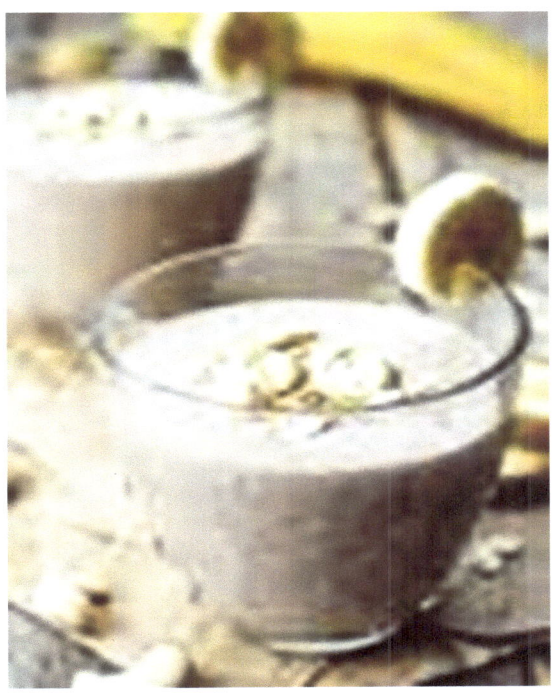

Banana is rich in potassium, which has heart-protective effects and aids in calcium absorption. This a great drink, which can help elevate energy. This is also a great protein drink to take before an intense workout. This protein smoothie will sustain muscle endurance and prevent cramps. This also maintains blood sugar to help you perform intense exercises longer.

Nutritional Facts:

Per 16-ounce serving:

- 499 calories
- 78 g carbohydrates
- 7 g fat
- 30 g protein
- 9 g fiber

Ingredients:

- 2 scoops protein powder vanilla-flavored
- 1 cup unsweetened almond milk
- 2 bananas
- 2 tablespoons rolled oats
- ½ cup cold water
- ¼ teaspoon cinnamon
- 1 teaspoon honey
- 4 ice cubes

To make:

Place all the ingredients in your blender, then blend until the mixture becomes smooth.

Berry Grape Protein Smoothie

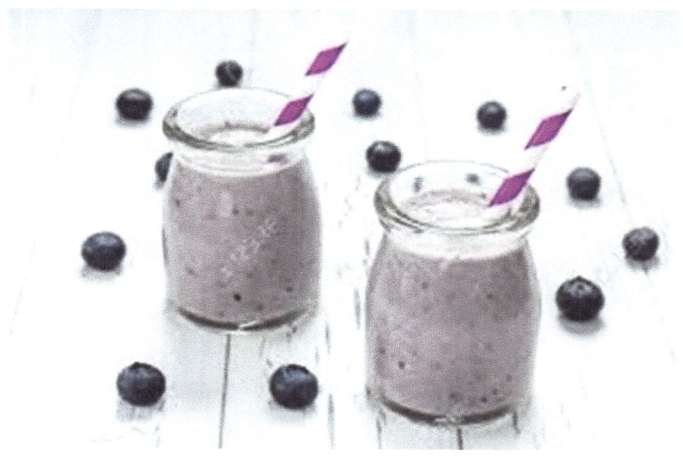

Plump juicy grapes give a good amount of Vitamin C, potassium and manganese. It is also full of powerful antioxidants that promote better health. Blending grapes in this smoothie recipe helps break down the skins, making the nutrients more available for the body to easily absorb.

Ingredients:

- 1 ½ cups of seedless grapes, red or purple variety
- 2 scoops of vanilla protein powder
- ½ cup of fresh blueberries
- 1 teaspoon of flaxseed oil
- 1 teaspoon of dry chia seeds
- ½ cup of water

To make:

Mix all the ingredients in a blender. Puree until smooth. Pour the smoothie in a serving glass. Serve. Sprinkle more chia seeds for added crunch and for garnish.

Nutritional Facts:

- 340 calories
- 43 g carbohydrates
- 9 g fiber
- 10 g fat
- 25 g protein

Peanut Butter and Chocolate Protein Smoothie

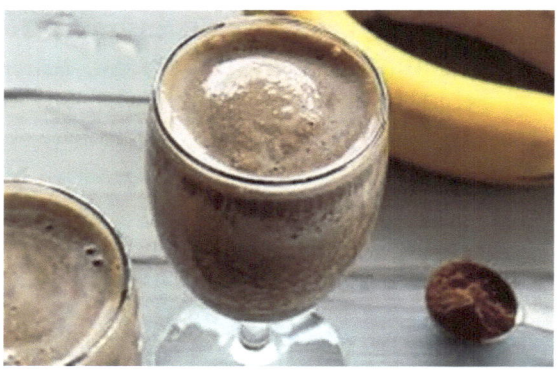

Chocolate and peanut butter is a powerful combination, which is not only delicious, but also good for your health. The goodness does not stop in the mouthwatering richness of chocolate and peanut butter. Peanuts are full of plant-based proteins that are good for you. It is also an excellent source of niacin, Vitamin E, manganese and folate. This is also a good source of monounsaturated fat and heart-supportive antioxidants. All that goodness packed in a small legume. Add the protein boost from the whey protein powder and you get an awesome protein-rich smoothie. Let's go to chocolate. Taste alone is more than enough reason to add chocolate to any food.

Aside from that, chocolate is rich in antioxidants and compounds that can improve every part of your body. Adding banana can further improve this drink. It gives a fruity surprise to the richness of peanut butter and chocolate. Its rich potassium content is a welcome addition to an already great list of nutrients.

Ingredients:

- 1 cup of dark chocolate, at least 70% cocoa

- 1 cup of unsweetened non-dairy milk, such as soy milk or almond milk
- 1 medium banana, sliced
- 2 tablespoons of peanut butter
- 3 to 5 ice cubes, adjusted according to preference

To make:

Place the ingredients in a blender. Adjust the amount of ice cube according to how you want your smoothie to taste. Pulse until well-blended. Pour in your glass, then serve immediately. If you want to make it even more delicious, add some chocolate shavings.

Nutritional Facts (for a 20-oz. serving):

- 485 calories
- 48 g carbohydrates
- 7 g fiber
- 21.5 g fat
- 32 g protein

Piña-Vocado Protein Smoothie

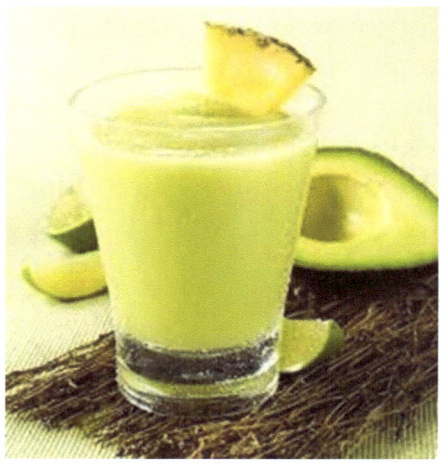

Pineapple is rich in phytonutrients that protect the heart from common problems such as atherosclerosis and heart attacks. It also helps lower cholesterol levels in the blood. Kale is rich in calcium, far more than what you get from a glass of cow's milk. It is also rich in healthy nutrients that benefit the body. Avocado is high in healthy fats that will help your tissues function better.

Ingredients:

- 1/3 cup of pineapple chunks
- ½ ripe avocado, diced
- 2 large handfuls (about 50 g) of kale leaves
- 2/3 cup of almond milk, unsweetened
- 1 scoop of vanilla protein powder
- 1 cup of ice cubes

To make:

Prepare all the ingredients and blend in your blender. Once the blender is smooth and creamy, pour the smoothie in a glass. Serve right away.

Nutritional Facts:

- 169 calories
- 6 g sugar
- 18 g protein

Chapter 4: Energy and Health Boosting Smoothie

Smoothies are can help you supply your body with all the nutrients that it needs in just a glass. This can be your go-to remedy when you need a quick energy boost any time of the day. Just one glass with the right ingredients and you will be at your top performance all day long.

Try these recipes to get your energy up. Not just that, these recipes will also help boost your health. Some of these recipes will strengthen your immunity, improve digestive functions, relieve stress and promote better overall health.

Chocolate Strawberry Indulgence Smoothie

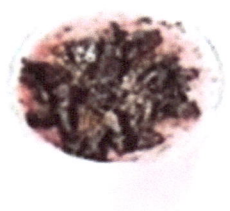

Chocolate is here again. For sure, nobody needs any more convincing if chocolate is involved. You get the PEA (phenylethylamine), which will boost your mood and increase your energy. You feel better and happier, so you get to do more. The antioxidants like theobromine will protect your cells from oxidative stress. This will help the cells work better because nothing hinders them. The cells get to produce more energy and use it more efficiently.

Adding strawberries enhances the flavor of this delicious smoothie. The slight acidity and tartness cuts the richness of chocolate just right.

Strawberries give important minerals and vitamins needed by your body. Beets add natural, low glycemic sweetness to the smoothie. Low glycemic means it does not cause the blood sugar levels to spike and crash, which is bad for the body. It is also rich in different minerals and vitamins that will support better health.

Ingredients:

- 1 tablespoon protein powder
- 2 teaspoons of raw cacao powder
- 1 ½ cups unsweetened almond milk
- 6 pieces of fresh strawberries
- ¼ cup of sliced beets
- 1 handful of spinach

To make:

Mix the ingredients in a blender on medium to high speed. Pour in a serving glass topped with sliced fresh strawberries.

Nutritional Facts:

- Calories 181.7
- Total fat (11.2%) 7.3 g
- Trans Fat (0.0%) 0.0 g
- Saturated Fat (2.3%) 0.5 g
- Cholesterol (0.0%) 0.0 mg
- Total Carbohydrates (5.3%) 15.8 g
- Dietary Fiber (24.5%) 6.1 g

- Sugars (0.0%) 3.5 g
- Protein 13.7 g
- Vitamin C 54.1%
- Vitamin E 2.1%
- Niacin 2.0%
- Thiamin 2.3%
- Folate 19.7%
- Iron 20.0%
- Panto. acid 1.0%
- Selenium 0.8%
- Magnesium 7.3%
- Manganese 22.2%
- Sodium 388.0 mg16.2%

Mood-Boosting Breakfast Smoothie

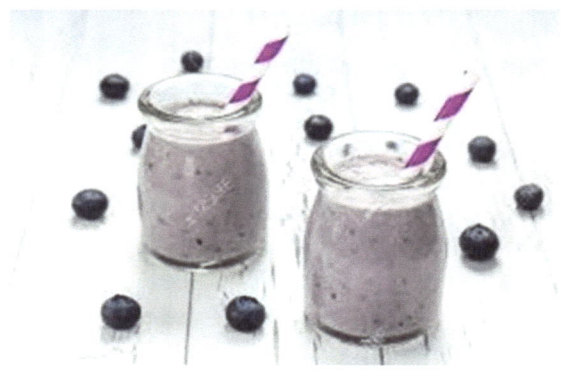

Depression is one of the leading reasons for low energy and poor performance. Lift your mood and increase your energy to accomplish what you need to do. You even get to have enough energy, so you can do the things you love.

This sweet smoothie is rich in nutrients that will provide longer lasting energy. Even though it's sweet, it will not produce a mid-morning crash. This recipe contains blueberries, banana and oats. Banana's potassium will help your muscles working well for hours. Oats will promote better cardiovascular health that will improve blood circulation. Good blood flow to the tissues will mean better blood supply to the brain, improving mood. Blueberries contain antioxidants that will help clear the systems of toxins that lead to poor mood and mental health.

Ingredients:

- ½ cup of oats
- ½ cup of walnuts
- 1 medium banana
- Handful of blueberries
- 1 cup of almond milk, unsweetened

To make:

Blend the ingredients in a blender on medium speed until smooth and creamy. Serve.

Nutritional Facts:

- Calories 477.2
- Total Carbohydrates 61.4 g
- Sugars 17.0 g
- Dietary Fiber 10.4 g
- Total fat 23.1 g
- Saturated Fat 2.0 g
- Sodium 256.3 mg
- Alcohol 0.0 g
- Protein 10.3 g
- Calcium 29.1%
- Vitamin D 0.0%
- Vitamin A 13.8%
- Vitamin K 11.4%

- Vitamin B6 27.8%
- Vitamin B12 0.0%
- Riboflavin 11.0%
- Phosphorus 27.4%
- Copper 31.4%
- Zinc 16.0%

Citrus Almond Smoothie

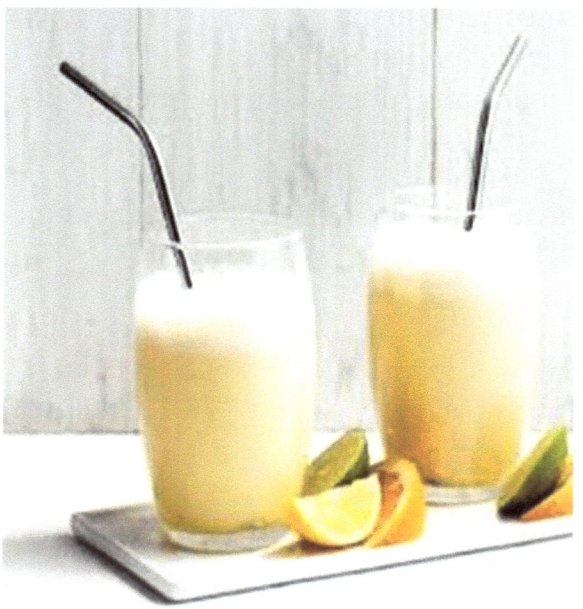

This smoothie recipe includes a great combination of citrus fruits that are rich in antioxidants and health-boosting nutrients. These can also raise your energy levels. Other health benefits include better sugar control, improved health and function of the heart, and reduced cholesterol levels.

Ingredients:

- 1 cup almond milk
- 1/2 cup freshly squeezed orange juice
- Juice from one lime
- Juice from one lemon
- 1 tablespoon honey
- Handful of ice

To make:

Mix all the ingredients in a blender until well combined and smooth. Pour in a serving glass and serve with a lime or lemon wedge.

Nutritional Facts:

- 148 calories
- 4 g fats (0 g saturated fat)
- 0 mg cholesterol
- 2 g fiber
- 29 g carbohydrates
- 2 g protein
- 191 mg sodium

Cucumber Celery Lime and Avocado Smoothie

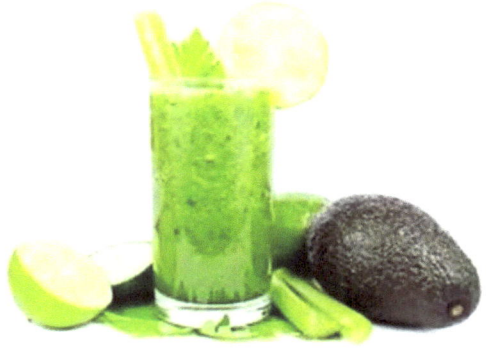

All the main ingredients of this smoothie can help boost your energy. The nutrients from all these can strengthen your immune system. Aside from that, it is also a refreshing drink that is sure to boost your energy for the day.

Ingredients:

- 1/8 medium avocado, sliced
- 1 medium celery stalk, diced
- ½ medium cucumber, sliced
- 2 tablespoon fresh lime juice
- 1 teaspoon agave nectar
- water to max line

To make:

Blend into a smooth consistency before pouring in a glass. Serve with a celery stalk and a lime wedge.

Nutritional Facts:

- Calories 105
- Total fat 5.2 g
- Total carbohydrates 15.8 g
- Sugars 8.9 g
- Dietary fiber 3.2 g
- Protein 1.8 g
- Sodium 37 mg

Chapter 5: Smoothie for Weight Loss

Weight loss is another benefit from regularly drinking a smoothie. Each smoothie is packed with nutrients needed by your body. It contains adequate amounts of proteins and fiber that make you feel full. Sugars are natural, thereby satisfying your cravings for sweets in a healthy way. These natural sugars do not cause spikes in blood glucose levels. These won't create unhealthy cravings that can increase your risk of developing diabetes and obesity.

Smoothies are also great if you want to keep meal portions under control. You can easily measure the ingredients, blend and pour in a glass. You won't likely reach for another serving and overeat if you stick to smoothies for meals.

Another way to get smoothies to help with weight loss is to use them to add more fiber and healthy proteins in your diet. These two nutrients are crucial in controlling your appetite.

So, you want to lose weight? Start including smoothies in your diet today. Begin your smoothie journey and start losing weight with these recipes.

Vanilla Almond Spinach and Mango Smoothie

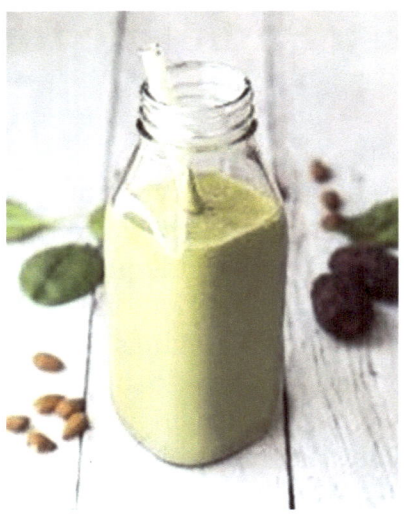

Vanilla is a good natural flavoring, which helps you feel satisfied with a meal - in this case, with a smoothie. You won't feel deprived or unsatisfied. That greatly helps in controlling portions and preventing cravings.

Spinach contains fiber and nutrients for proper body nutrition even when you are trying to lose weight. Mangoes add to the vitamin and mineral content of the smoothie, further improving the nutrition you get from each serving. Almond butter and almond milk give a protein boost that will help you build lean muscles. This is important when trying to lose weight.

Ingredients:

- 1 cup almond milk
- 2 tablespoon almond butter
- ½ cup spinach leaves
- 1 splash of vanilla extract
- ½ cup of mangoes

To make:

Blend into a smooth mixture in a blender on high speed. Pour into a serving glass and enjoy.

Nutritional Facts:

- Calories 415.5
- Total carbohydrates 8.3% RDA (24.8 g)
- Dietary Fiber 31.0% (7.7 g)
- Sugars 0.0% (13.0 g)
- Total fat 37.4% (24.3 g)
- Saturated Fat 7.1% (1.4 g)
- Sodium 15.5% (373.1 mg)
- Protein 29.8 g
- Vitamin C 57.1%
- Vitamin A 54.0%
- Vitamin D 0.0%
- Vitamin K 94.9%
- Vitamin E 29.3%
- Thiamin 3.2%
- Niacin 8.4%
- Riboflavin 21.3%
- Vitamin B6 8.0%
- Vitamin B12 0.0%
- Folate 20.4%
- Pantothenic acid 2.7%
- Calcium 33.5%
- Phosphorus 18.2%
- Iron 29.2%
- Magnesium 27.4%
- Selenium 2.0%
- Zinc 8.1%
- Manganese 43.7%

- Copper 20.6%

PB & J Smoothie

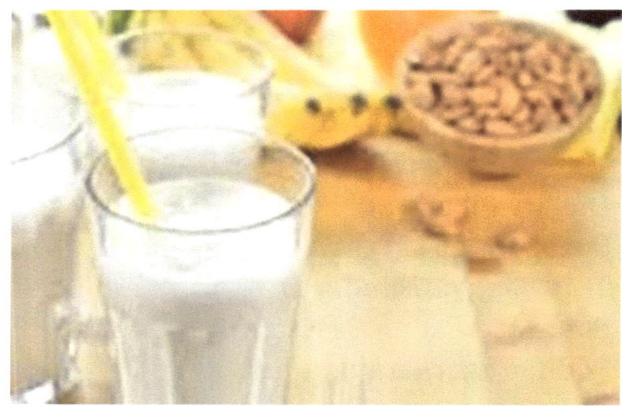

Peanut butter and jelly is not limited to a sandwich. You can still enjoy this favorite in a smoothie. This is perfect when you are trying to lose weight.

Peanut butter is a rich source of proteins that help build lean muscles. This helps your body focus more on burning fats rather than in slowing down metabolism in an attempt to slow down muscle wasting. The "jelly" part of this PB & J smoothie can be attributed to the addition of yogurt, banana and strawberries. This combination produces that fruity, creamy, sweet goodness of jelly that perfectly complements with peanut butter.

Banana is rich in potassium and other nutrients that can boost metabolism and promote weight loss. It is also filling, helping you control appetite and cravings. Strawberries give a sweet yet tart flavor that can help you satisfy your sweet tooth. This can also help you deal with cravings that can otherwise derail your weight loss journey. Yogurt is full of probiotics that improve digestion.

Better digestive function helps promote better metabolism and weight loss.

Ingredients:

- 4 ounces nonfat Greek yogurt, plain
- 2 teaspoons plain peanut butter
- 2 cups fresh or frozen strawberries, sliced
- 1 frozen banana, sliced
- 1/2 cup ice

To make:

Blend into a smooth and creamy, delicious smoothie in a blender on high speed. Place in a glass and serve garnished with half a strawberry.

Nutrition facts:

- Calories 327
- Carbohydrates 55 g
- Fiber 9 g
- Protein 18 g
- Fat 7 g (1.4 g saturated fat)
- Sodium 94 mg

Tropical Breakfast Smoothie

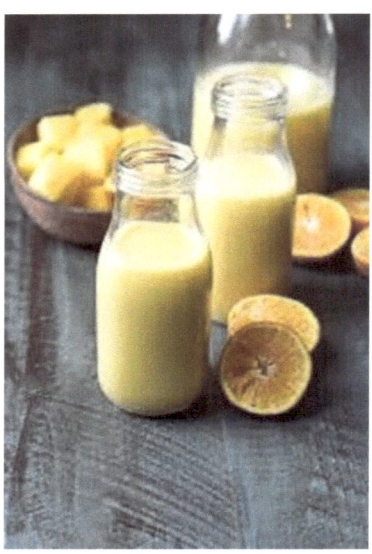

This is a great way to start your day with a power-packed, refreshing smoothie. This recipe will give you a vitamin boost that will surely rev up your metabolism.

Yogurt will give a good dose of probiotics to get your digestive system working properly. Mango will give vitamins and minerals, along with phytonutrients that support fat burning and better metabolism.

Ingredients:

- 6 ounces nonfat plain Greek yogurt
- 1/2 cup fresh pineapple, diced
- 1/2 cup frozen or fresh mango, sliced
- 1 fresh or frozen banana, sliced
- 2 tablespoons of ground flaxseed

To make:

Puree the ingredients in a blender on medium speed. Once smooth and well mixed, pour the smoothie in a glass and serve.

Nutritional Facts:

- 368 calories
- 60 g carbohydrate
- 9 g fiber
- 22 g protein
- 7 g fat (0.9 g saturated fats)
- 68 mg sodium

Sweet Spinach Smoothie

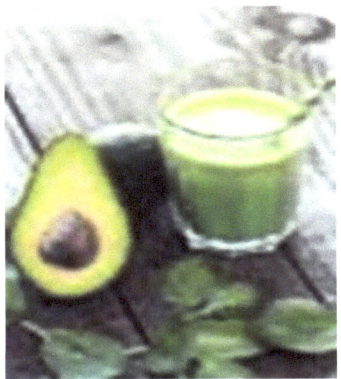

Spinach is a nutritious leafy vegetable you should consider adding to your weight loss smoothies. It is rich in fiber, which can control appetite. It is also full of nutrients that will support a healthy metabolism.

Grapes and pear will give this smoothie a sweetness to satisfy your sweet tooth. Do not worry, the sugar these fruits give are of the healthy kind. It won't cause sugar crashes and intensify cravings. In fact, these natural sugars can stabilize your blood glucose levels, so you won't experience low energy. This will greatly help you avoid reaching for unhealthy, fattening snacks.

Avocado is rich in healthy fats. This helps you feel full and satisfied with just a glass of this delicious smoothie. You won't be overeating with this smoothie. Lime juice gives a boost of Vitamin C to the blend. This can rev up your metabolism and detoxifies your body for enhanced weight loss.

Ingredients:

- 2 cups (packed) spinach leaves
- 6 ounces nonfat Greek yogurt, plain
- 1 ripe medium pear, peel and core removed, then sliced
- 2 tablespoons diced avocado
- 15 pieces of red or green grapes
- 1-2 tablespoons lime juice, freshly squeezed

To make:

- 316 calories
- 52 g carbohydrate
- 9 g fiber
- 21 g protein
- 6 g fat (0.9 g saturated fats)
- 115 mg sodium

Conclusion

Thank you for purchasing this book.

Congratulations! Now that you have finished this book, you are equipped with the tools that you need to live a healthier life and lose weight with smoothies. The recipes are so easy to make. You don't have to learn new kitchen skills. Just place the fruits and vegetables in a blender, add water or milk, blend and pour in your glass. You get all the goodness of fresh fruits and vegetables in a convenient way.

Start making smoothies right now and experience the health benefits.

Good luck on your journey to a healthier, leaner new you.

www.ingramcontent.com/pod-product-compliance
Lightning Source LLC
Chambersburg PA
CBHW050755290526
45792CB00008B/2188